GREATER MEKONG SUBREGION HEALTH COOPERATION STRATEGY 2024–2030

DECEMBER 2024

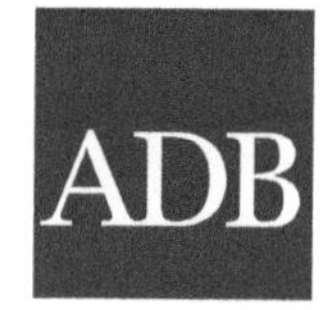

ASIAN DEVELOPMENT BANK

CONTENTS

TABLE, FIGURES, AND BOXES

ABBREVIATIONS

ADB	–	Asian Development Bank
AMR	–	antimicrobial resistance
APHSAF	–	Asia Pacific Health Security Action Framework
ASEAN	–	Association of Southeast Asian Nations
CDC	–	Communicable Disease Control
GDP	–	gross domestic product
GMS	–	Greater Mekong Subregion
GMS-2030	–	Greater Mekong Subregion Economic Cooperation Program Strategic Framework 2030
HCS	–	Health Cooperation Strategy
IHR	–	International Health Regulations
Lao PDR	–	Lao People's Democratic Republic
PHC	–	primary health care
PRC	–	People's Republic of China
RAI	–	Regional Artemisinin-Resistance Initiative
RCI	–	regional cooperation and integration
RIF	–	Regional Investment Framework
SDG	–	Sustainable Development Goal
UHC	–	universal health coverage
WGHC	–	Working Group on Health Cooperation
WHO	–	World Health Organization

EXECUTIVE SUMMARY

The *Greater Mekong Subregion Health Cooperation Strategy 2024–2030* (HCS 2024–2030) reaffirms the direction of its precursor, the first *Greater Mekong Subregion Health Cooperation Strategy 2019–2023*. It aligns with the *Greater Mekong Subregion Economic Cooperation Program (GMS Program) Strategic Framework 2030 (GMS-2030)*.

In the Greater Mekong Subregion (GMS), regional health cooperation leverages the subregion's expertise in health leadership, human resources, and programmatic experience to address common health challenges. Consistent with the GMS Program's mandate, it focuses on health issues that are regional in nature and require collective action to address. The strategy will guide programming, foster innovation, increase engagement with the development and private sector partners, and mobilize new financing to support its implementation. It has two strategic pillars: regional health security and health system strengthening toward universal health coverage (UHC). Its crosscutting themes are gender, climate change, and digital health.

HCS 2024–2030 builds on a 2-decades long history of support from development partners to strengthen regional cooperation in health. The GMS Working Group on Health Cooperation (WGHC) with the Asian Development Bank (ADB) as its Secretariat serves as a platform for addressing regional health challenges. It facilitates dialogue and supports the development of policies, strategies, and programmatic responses.

The HCS 2024–2030 will look for opportunities for cross-sector collaboration where there are significant common development benefits to health and other sectors. Leveraging the knowledge, technical resources, and capital of the private sector and development partners will be critical to achieving the ambitious health targets of the GMS countries.

I INTRODUCTION

The Greater Mekong Subregion (GMS) comprises Cambodia, Yunnan Province and Guangxi Zhuang Autonomous Region in the People's Republic of China (PRC), the Lao People's Democratic Republic (Lao PDR), Myanmar, Thailand, and Viet Nam.[1] The GMS is a naturally interconnected economic region defined by the Mekong River and is home to around 326 million people. Regional health cooperation is a key priority for the GMS countries, and an integral part of the GMS Economic Cooperation Program (GMS Program)[2] Strategic Framework 2030 (GMS-2030).[3]

GMS-2030 provides a framework for subregional collaboration "on seven long-term, powerful trends: (i) risk of pandemics; (ii) weaker global growth and the threat to free trade; (iii) persistent pockets of poverty and increasing in-country inequality; (iv) severe environmental challenges and threats from climate change, disaster events, and pollution; (v) technological change and digitalization; (vi) evolving demographics; and (vii) rapid urbanization" (footnote 3).

GMS-2030 is underpinned by three pillars: community, connectivity, and competitiveness, and will strengthen the commitment made under the previous GMS Strategic Framework 2012–2022 to scale up interventions under pillar 1, the community pillar. It aims to build a greater sense of community and promote the development of a healthy and environmentally sustainable GMS in which the well-being of all citizens is pursued (footnote 3). GMS-2030 also aims to identify shared approaches for addressing regional health issues and explore ways to augment resources allocated to regional health initiatives. The *Greater Mekong Subregion Health Cooperation Strategy 2024–2030* (henceforth HCS 2024–2030) will be a vehicle to help achieve this.

Efforts to advance regional cooperation and integration (RCI), which are crucial drivers for economic growth, expose the GMS to distinct health challenges. Highly mobile populations—both cross-border migration and displaced populations—impact health systems and disease control efforts. For example, migrants, who are a key workforce and a driver of economic development in the GMS, face health challenges at various stages of their migration journey and are at risk of becoming marginalized and

---

[1] ADB has placed a temporary hold on sovereign project disbursements and new contracts in Myanmar effective 1 February 2021.

[2] The GMS Economic Cooperation Program aims to promote regional cooperation, economic development, and poverty reduction in the Greater Mekong Subregion. It is an inclusive program of partners including multilateral development banks, bilateral partners, private sector, nongovernment organizations, and governments. The program started in 1992 and its investment and technical assistance projects have reached 30.3 billion (source: Greater Mekong Subregion. Six Nations Three Decades One Vision).

[3] ADB. 2021. *The Greater Mekong Subregion (GMS) Economic Cooperation Program Strategic Framework 2030* (GMS-2030).

excluded from essential health care. Access to essential health services, including disease prevention, along with surveillance and early warning mechanisms are critical to health security and human capital development.[4]

Regional health cooperation offers an opportunity to utilize the subregion's expertise in health leadership, human resource capabilities, and programmatic experience to tackle the shared health issues. The first GMS Health Cooperation Strategy 2019–2023 acknowledged the significant track record of collaboration among GMS countries in addressing those health challenges. Its vision, objectives, and key activities responded to the priorities identified during extensive consultations and were consistent with national health plans.[5]

The HCS 2024–2030 focuses on health issues that are regional in nature and require collective action to address. Setting out the strategic and operational priorities for regional health cooperation over 7 years, this new strategy also reinforces and reaffirms the direction of its precursor, the Greater Mekong Subregion Health Cooperation Strategy 2019–2023. The lessons learned during the pandemic were instrumental in its formation. Similarly, consultations with the members of the GMS Working Group on Health Cooperation (WGHC), governments, the private sector, and other development partners at both country and regional levels informed its development. The strategy reflects the countries' priorities and is aligned with the GMS 2030 Mission Statement,[6] the national health plans in each country, and the Ha Noi Declaration on the Initiative for ASEAN Integration.[7] The HCS 2024–2030 also considers the central and special role migration plays, and the challenges posed by climate change. Lastly, it aims to increase engagement with the private sector to find innovative solutions to the region's health challenges.

The HCS 2024–2030 will help resolve regional health challenges and gaps by mitigating the ongoing threats and risks linked to health security and climate change, addressing some of the regulatory and policy challenges, and supporting regional public goods, such as UHC and workforce development. It has two strategic pillars—*regional health security and health system strengthening toward UHC*—which are aligned with defined programming areas (Figure 1).

---

[4]   World Health Organization. 2024. *Asia Pacific Health Security Action Framework*.
[5]   ADB. 2019. Greater Mekong Subregion Health Cooperation Strategy 2019–2023.
[6]   The GMS 2030 Mission Statement calls for embracing the three core principles of (i) environmental sustainability and resilience, (ii) internal and external integration, and (iii) inclusivity (including equitable human capital development) (footnote 3).
[7]   ASEAN. 2020. *Ha Noi Declaration on the Adoption of the Initiative for ASEAN Integration (2021-2025)*.

Figure 1: Strategic Framework of the Greater Mekong Subregion Health Cooperation Strategy 2024–2030

Vision: Through collective efforts, we aim to foster a healthy and sustainable GMS community, where the well-being of all citizens is pursued

Outcomes	Improved GMS health system performance in preparing for and responding to all hazards and acute public health threats	Decreased disparities in health care access among different vulnerable groups	
Pillars	Regional health security	Health system strengthening toward UHC	Crosscutting
Programming Areas	IHR core capacities Antimicrobial resistance Strengthen CDC cross-border cooperation	Access to health products Health workforce and infrastructure development Service delivery for all (including migrant, older people and other vulnerable groups)	Gender
Indicative Activities	• Strengthen governance and regulatory infrastructure for emergency-use therapeutics and vaccines • Explore strategic regional stockpiles for essential medical equipment and vaccines • Strengthen and utilize regional AMR networks • Collaborate to study AMR trends, transmission pathways, and innovative solutions • Enhance cross-border CDC coordination through health emergency simulation exercises and drills • Strengthen the regional digital platform for sharing critical health information, early warning, and surveillance data	• Explore pooled procurement or public and private collaborations to increase the availability and affordability of health products, including vaccines and pharmaceuticals • Provide targeted opportunities for health workforce development (e.g., FETP Thailand) • Establish and operationalize GMS centers of excellence or collaboration • Showcase the work of the WGHC • Improve migrant health (e.g., extending access to essential health services, policy coherence, and promoting financial risk protection) • Develop processes for mutual recognition of qualifications and collaborative training programs	Climate change Digital heatlh

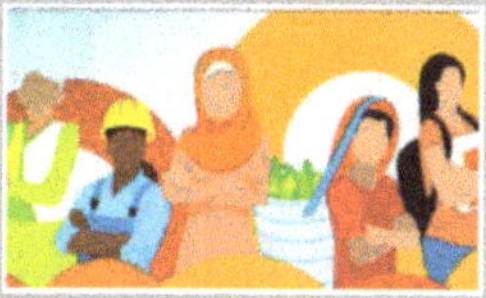

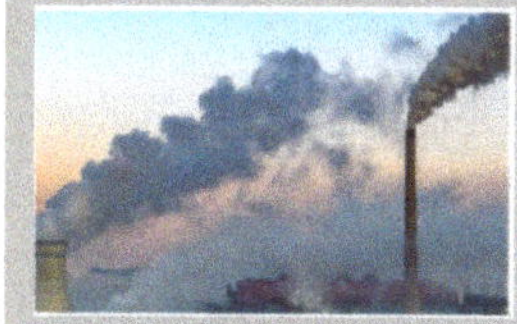

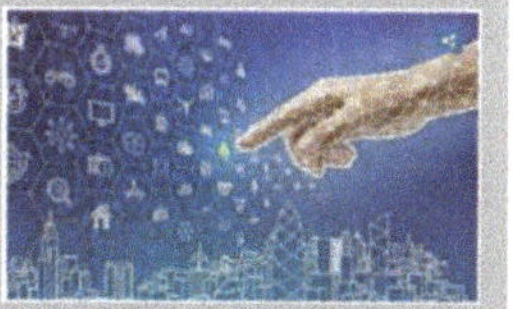

AMR = antimicrobial resistance, CDC = communicable disease control, FETP = field epidemiology training program, GMS = Greater Mekong Subregion, IHR = International Health Regulations, UHC = universal health coverage, WGHC = Working Group on Health Cooperation.
Source: Asian Development Bank.

BACKGROUND

Health Challenges

Over the last 2 decades, the GMS has witnessed notable advancements in health indicators, reflecting the collective efforts to address public health challenges. Improvements have been observed in life expectancy, maternal and child health, and infectious diseases. Enhanced health care infrastructure, increased access to essential health services, and collaborative regional initiatives have contributed to these positive trends. The GMS countries have demonstrated resilience in the face of emerging health threats and have implemented effective strategies to mitigate them, although challenges continue. Persistent disparities in health outcomes and service coverage by ethnicity, income quintile, gender, and geography remain. Not all population groups across the GMS are benefiting equally from the improvements.

Among the challenges faced by the GMS are rising rates of chronic diseases, an aging population, and the need for sustained efforts to ensure equitable access to health care. For example, the proportion of people aged over 60 years in the PRC is expected to increase from 12% in 2010 to 33% by 2050, making its population the oldest in the world.[8] By 2011, Viet Nam had one of the highest rates of older people in the world, but its health care system has not yet adapted. Purpose-built health care facilities and appropriate levels of skilled health care workers for older people are lacking. Continued regional cooperation, investment in health care systems including infrastructure, and a focus on primary health care are crucial to further advance health indicators and foster a healthier future in GMS countries.

The GMS frequently experiences public health emergencies caused by infectious diseases; antimicrobial resistance (AMR); food safety incidents; and climate change and extreme weather events, including floods.[9] The impact of these emergencies leads to a wide range of negative economic, health, and social impacts, including increased morbidity and mortality, disruption to health care delivery, school closures, food insecurity, and loss of income. Public health emergencies impose additional economic burdens due to business closures, response efforts, and lost productivity from illness (footnote 4). For instance, over the past 20 years, GMS countries have faced several outbreaks of avian influenza in poultry, both with and without epidemiological links to human infections. These outbreaks have led to extensive poultry culling and caused substantial financial losses to households and the poultry industry.[10]

---

[8] ADB. 2014. Challenges and Opportunities of Population Aging in the People's Republic of China.

[9] World Health Organization Regional Office for the Western Pacific. 2017. *Asia Pacific Strategy for Emerging Diseases and Public Health Emergencies (APSED III): Advancing Implementation of the International Health Regulations (2005)*.

[10] A. Suttie et al. 2019. Avian Influenza in the Greater Mekong Subregion, 2003–2018. *Infection, Genetics and Evolution*. Vol. 74.

The Coronavirus Disease 2019 Pandemic

The health care systems, medical resources, and personnel were strained by the coronavirus disease pandemic in unprecedented ways. The challenges included managing a high number of cases and new processes for border closures and quarantine, supply-chain interference, and implementation of multi-age vaccination programs. The pandemic disrupted essential health services and routine immunization, leading to a reversal of gains in many areas. In the third round of the World Health Organization (WHO) Global Pulse Survey on the continuity of essential health services during the pandemic, over 90% of the countries surveyed reported ongoing disruptions to essential health services.[11] A 2022 *Lancet* study found a higher level of service disruption than reported in WHO Global Pulse Survey estimates.[12]

In the GMS, some examples of service disruption included, in the Lao PDR, the coverage rate of fully immunized children fell from 76.3% in 2019 to 68.6% in 2022.[13] In Thailand, the government repurposed hospitals to serve as specific treatment centers, causing a delay in elective surgeries and routine treatments. In Cambodia, disruptions to HIV care services led to a loss of access to HIV treatments and delays in viral load testing.[14] In other parts of Southeast Asia, progress in reproductive, maternal, neonatal, and child health outcomes slowed or worsened for the first time in decades (footnote 12).

The GMS Program's COVID-19 Response and Recovery Plan 2021–2023 sought to coordinate the efforts of GMS countries on issues that needed enhanced RCI for an effective pandemic response. The plan complemented national efforts by concentrating on RCI priorities to (i) harmonize health, economic, environmental, and social objectives; (ii) involve the private sector; (iii) include local governments and communities; and (iv) ensure extensive and effective communication.[15] ADB assistance to the GMS countries during the pandemic totalled $2,310 million, which included six GMS health projects.[16]

Beyond the health sector, the pandemic affected various areas, including significant drops in domestic demand, reduced tourism and business travel, disruptions in trade and production links, and supply chain interruptions. Being heavily dependent on cross-border travel and tourism, GMS countries were severely affected (Table).

---

[11] WHO. 2022. Essential Health Services Face Continued Disruption During COVID-19 Pandemic.

[12] T. Gadsden et al. 2024. Impact of COVID-19 on Essential Service Provision for Reproductive, Maternal, Neonatal, and Child Health in the Southeast Asia Region: A Systematic Review. *The Lancet Regional Health—Southeast Asia.* Vol. 25.

[13] World Bank. 2023. *Project Appraisal Document for Health and Nutrition Services Access Project Phase II.*

[14] K. Seang et al. 2023. Using Relational Community Engagement within the Digital Health Intervention (DHI) to Improve Access and Retention among People Living with HIV (PLWH): Findings from a Mixed-Method Study in Cambodia. *Int J Environ Res Public Health.* 20 (7). p. 5247.

[15] ADB. 2021. The Greater Mekong Subregion COVID-19 Response and Recovery Plan 2021–2023.

[16] The six GMS projects include (i) The Cambodia Border Areas Health Project (53290-001), (ii) The Lao PDR Border Areas Health Project (53290-002), (iii) The Cambodia Rapid Immunization Support Project under the Asia Pacific Vaccine Access Facility (55104-001), (iv) Additional Financing to the GMS Health Security Project in Cambodia (48118-002), (v) Additional financing to the GMS Health Security Project in the Lao PDR (48118-003), (vi) Additional financing to the GMS Health Security Project in Myanmar (48118-004). Noting the Myanmar project was approved by the ADB Board, but did not proceed as ADB placed a temporary hold on sovereign project disbursements and new contracts in Myanmar effective 1 February 2021.

Table: Decline in Tourism Revenues in the Greater Mekong Subregion

Country	Best Case		Moderate Case		Worse Case	
	Share in GDP (%)	Amount ($ million)	Share in GDP (%)	Amount ($ million)	Share in GDP (%)	Amount ($ million)
Cambodia	–1.409	–345.7	–1.929	–473.4	–3.490	–856.5
Thailand	–0.845	–4,265.8	–1.224	–6,180.2	–2.361	–11,923.5
Viet Nam	–0.432	–1,059.2	–0.164	–1,504.6	–1.158	–2,840.6
Myanmar	–0.149	–1,06.3	–0.224	–159.4	–0.448	–318.8
Lao People's Democratic Republic	–0.164	–29.5	–0.231	–41.5	–431.000	–77.4
People's Republic of China	–0.112	–15,241.6	–0.149	–20,215.0	–0.258	–35,135.3

– means decrease.
GDP = gross domestic product.
Source: Estimates from ADB. 2020. The Economic Impact of the COVID-19 Outbreak on Developing Asia.

The effects of public health emergencies extend well beyond the health sector, highlighting the interconnectedness of health, economics, and society, and the potential for such events to trigger wider crises. Health security systems that aim to prevent or mitigate the effects of these emergencies play a crucial role in maintaining broader socioeconomic stability and advancing development goals. The Asia Pacific Health Security Action Framework (APHSAF) advocates for a comprehensive approach, involving both government and societal engagement to effectively address the public health impacts of emergencies. It requires the involvement of all government sectors and agencies, as well as all relevant stakeholders, to enhance community resilience and integrate health security into pertinent national and local policies and practices (footnote 4).

Responding to the pandemic provided useful insights and valuable lessons for the GMS countries and helped them to strengthen their health systems ahead of another pandemic. Preparedness needs a robust and resilient health system, particularly in primary care, to detect disease outbreaks, deliver essential health care services, and support the distribution of public health interventions. Ongoing efforts to support health security and strengthen national health systems, to enable universal health coverage (UHC)[17] are essential for that preparedness.

In a 2021 evaluation, ADB assessed the performance and results of the GMS Program during 2012–2020, and stated that the pandemic underscored the heightened necessity and significance of regional cooperation mechanisms like the GMS Program. These platforms, it suggested, were essential for fostering policy discussions and communication between neighboring nations, facilitating trade, enhancing cooperation among border authorities, and bolstering collaboration across national boundaries. ADB likewise stated that the lessons learned from the pandemic emphasize the importance of fostering GMS health cooperation to prepare for similar events in the future.[18]

---

[17]   Universal health coverage provides access for everyone to a complete range of quality health services that they need, when and where they need them, and without financial hardship.
[18]   ADB. 2021. Evaluation of ADB Support for the Greater Mekong Subregion Program, 2012–2020.

Lessons from the Previous Strategy

The review of the GMS Health Cooperation Strategy 2019–2023 conducted in May 2023 recommended the following six actions to be addressed during the implementation of the HCS 2024–2030.

(i)   increase the use of partnership agreements for improved cross-border health collaborations;

(ii)   improve the support from the WGHC and its Secretariat (ADB) to advance health cooperation and to build a stronger portfolio of health projects in the GMS;

(iii)   establish a technical advisory group or task force to support the technical activities of the WGHC and a specific focal point to oversee each strategic pillar;

(iv)   encourage opportunities for increased cross-sector collaboration and intragovernmental promotion of the strategy and engagement with the private sector;

(v)   develop deeper mechanisms and increase technical support for monitoring and evaluation at regional and national levels; and

(vi)   develop capacity-building initiatives and training programs particularly in leadership and governance.

Strategy Development Process and Alignment

The HCS 2024–2030 uses the successes of the GMS Program and ambition of GMS-2030 to tackle increasingly complex issues. It will guide programming; foster innovation; increase engagement from development partners, the private sector, and civil society; as well as mobilize new project financing to support results. In addition to GMS-2030 and the APHSAF (footnotes 3 and 4), several global and regional policies have informed this strategy, including the following:

(i)   One Health High-Level Panel policy;[19]

(ii)   One Health Joint Plan of Action (2022–2026);[20]

(iii)   Post-2015 Health Development Agenda of the Association of Southeast Asian Nations 2021–2025;[21]

(iv)   Paris Agreement;[22]

[19]   WHO. 2023. One Health High-Level Expert Panel.
[20]   FAO et al. 2022. One Health Joint Plan of Action, 2022–2026—Working Together for the Health of Humans, Animals, Plants and the Environment.
[21]   ASEAN. 2023. ASEAN's Post-2015 Health Development Agenda (2021–2025).
[22]   Paris Agreement to the United Nations Framework Convention on Climate Change. 2015. T.I.A.S. No. 16-1104.

(v)   United Nations General Assembly High-Level Meeting on Pandemic Prevention, Preparedness and Response;[23]

(vi)   United Nations Sustainable Development Goals (SDGs);[24]

(vii)   Global Health Security Index;[25]

(viii) WHO International Health Regulations (2005);[26] and

(ix)   WHO 14th General Programme of Work (GPW 14).[27]

The HCS 2024–2030 builds on efforts by GMS countries and the Association of Southeast Asian Nations (ASEAN) to develop a more cohesive regional response to future health crises. Key health security initiatives, such as the ASEAN Emergency Operations Centre Network for public health emergencies, the ASEAN Joint Multi-Sectoral Outbreak Investigation and Response System, and the ASEAN-Plus Three Field Epidemiology Training Network, are helping to jointly prepare for and address public health emergencies.[28]

All GMS countries are signatories to the Paris Agreement on climate change,[29] the Sendai Framework for Disaster Risk Reduction,[30] and the 2030 Agenda for SDG (footnote 26). The 2024 Sustainable Development Report provides a global evaluation of countries' progress in achieving the SDGs. It complements the official SDG indicators and voluntary national reviews and considers the performance of each country against specific SDGs. Across the GMS, progress was mixed. Most countries were seen to have "major" remaining challenges, and all were seen to not be "improving sufficiently to attain the goal for SDG 3" (Good Health and Well-Being).[31] Voluntary submission of their national reports for the Midterm Review of the Implementation of the Sendai Framework has been completed by Cambodia, the Lao PDR, Thailand, and Viet Nam.[32]

The 2021 Global Health Security Index found that despite considerable efforts to respond to the pandemic, countries including in the GMS, still lacked adequate readiness to confront future epidemics and pandemics. Structured around six categories, the Index is designed to evaluate a country's capacity to prevent, detect, and manage biological threats. It scored the GMS countries (and the difference from the 2019 Index) as follows: Cambodia 31.1 (+0.1), the Lao PDR 34.8 (+2.0), the PRC 47.5 (–1.5), Thailand 68.2 (–0.7), and Viet Nam 42.9 (+0.7) (footnote 25).

---

[23]   UN General Assembly. Preparing for the UN High-Level Meeting on Pandemic Prevention, Preparedness and Response, 2023.

[24]   United Nations. Sustainable Development Goals.

[25]   J. A. Bell and J. B. Nuzzo. 2021. *Global Health Security Index: Advancing Collective Action and Accountability Amid Global Crisis* (accessed 12 December 2023).

[26]   WHO. 2024. *International Health Regulations (2005) as Amended in 2014 and 2022*. See para. 30 on expected changes to IHR (2005).

[27]   WHO. Fourteenth General Programme of Work.

[28]   These regional initiatives will be augmented by the ASEAN Centres for Public Health Emergencies and Emerging Diseases.

[29]   United Nations. List of Parties That Signed the Paris Agreement on 22 April 2016.

[30]   The framework outlines four key action priorities: (i) improving the understanding of disaster risk; (ii) bolstering disaster risk governance to manage these risks; (iii) investing in disaster risk reduction to build resilience; and (iv) enhancing preparedness for effective disaster response, recovery, rehabilitation, and reconstruction efforts.

[31]   J. D. Sachs et al. 2024. *Implementing the SDG Stimulus. Sustainable Development Report 2024.*

[32]   UNDRR. Midterm Review of the Sendai Framework for Disaster Risk Reduction 2015–2030.

National Health Systems and Priorities

The health systems in GMS countries differ structurally, and their operational history, coverage, and quality vary, but they do share a range of common health system concerns. These include (i) achieving UHC; (ii) strengthening disease control; (iii) building and upgrading infrastructure, particularly in rural and underserved areas; (v) health system strengthening, which includes capacity building the workforce, supply chain management, and information systems; (vi) developing and enhancing disaster preparedness and response capabilities; and (vii) reducing health disparities to ensure equitable access to services, especially for marginalized and vulnerable populations, including older people (Box 1).

Box 1: Strategic Health Plans of Countries in the Greater Mekong Subregion

Each country in the Greater Mekong Subregion (GMS) has a strategic health plan providing a structured and organized approach to improving health care systems and services. These plans guide decision-making, resource allocation, and health system goals.

- In Cambodia, the fourth Health Strategic Plan, 2024–2033 is in the final stages of development. Its goal is "improved equitable health outcomes and enhanced financial protection" with four strategic objectives. It commits to continuing to advance the national health development agenda, ensuring it promotes healthy lives and well-being for all at all ages.[a]

- In Thailand, the 20-year National Strategic Plan for Public Health 2017–2036 is intended to provide guidance for public health agencies to develop and implement a health system that is in line with the national policy, and with the health system reform agenda of "Thailand achieving security and prosperity and becoming a developed nation based on the philosophy of self-sufficiency economy."[b]

- In the Lao People's Democratic Republic, the Health Sector Reform Strategy and Framework (2013–2025) is set out in four phases. Its goal is to establish an effective health care system ensuring improving quality of health care services, achieving universal health coverage for all, and protecting and promoting the health of the people.[c]

- In Viet Nam, the Ministry of Health approved a new national strategy in 2024 to protect, care for, and improve people's health in the period to 2030, with a vision of the people enjoying the best medical services to 2045.[d]

- In the People's Republic of China, the national strategy Healthy China 2030 is a plan that guides Yunnan Province and Guangxi Zhuang Autonomous Region, and places a high priority on enhancing the quality of primary health care in rural areas by leveraging innovations and health system efficiencies.[e]

---

[a] Ministry of Health. 2023. Outline of the Health Strategic Plan 2024–2033 Working Together for the Future: A Safer and Healthier Cambodia. Paper presented at the National Health Congress, February 2023, Phnom Penh.
[b] Government of Thailand. 2017. 20-Year National Strategic Plan for Public Health 2017–2036. Ministry of Public Health.
[c] Ministry of Health of the Lao People's Democratic Republic. 2022. Health Sector Reform Strategy (2021–2030). Vientiane.
[d] Trích yêu: Quyêt đinh Phê duyêt Chiên lúôc quôc gia bão vê, chăm sóc và nâng cao súc khóe nhân dân giai đoan đên năm 2030, tâm nhìn đên năm 2045 [Decision Approving the National Strategy to Protect, Care for and Improve People's Health in the Period to 2030, with a Vision to 2045].
[e] Government of the People's Republic of China. 2016. The Healthy China 2030. State Council.
Source: Asian Development Bank.

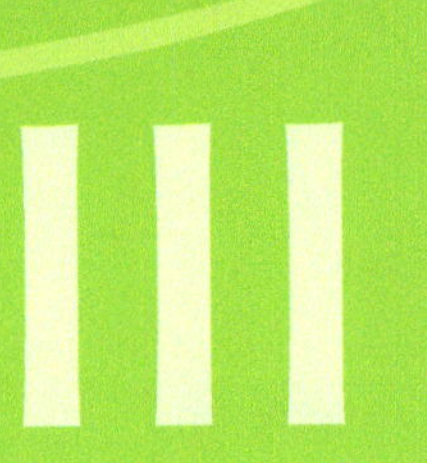

III THE GREATER MEKONG SUBREGION HEALTH COOPERATION STRATEGY 2024–2030

Vision and Outcomes

The vision for the HCS 2024–2030 is aligned with GMS-2030. Central to its attainment are two outcomes also aligned with the GMS-2030 and with the GMS-2030 Results Framework (Box 2).[33]

> ### Box 2: Vision and Outcomes of the Greater Mekong Subregion Health Cooperation Strategy 2024–2030
>
> The vision for the Greater Mekong Subregion (GMS) Health Cooperation Strategy 2024–2030 (HCS 2024-2030) is "Through collective efforts, we aim to foster a healthy and sustainable GMS community, where the well-being of all citizens is pursued."
>
> The two outcomes of the HCS 2024–2030 are:
>
> - Improved GMS health system performance in preparing for and responding to all hazards, and acute public health threats.
>
> - Decreased disparities in health care access among different vulnerable groups.
>
> Source: Asian Development Bank.

Strategic Framework

This HCS 2024–2030 sets out the strategic and operational priorities for regional health cooperation in the next 7 years. It contains two strategic pillars—*regional health security and health system strengthening toward UHC*—which are aligned with outcomes. Each pillar has defined programming areas representing some of the possible operational priorities for GMS health cooperation. These areas will shape future projects and activities (Figure 1).

---

[33] ADB. 2022. *Greater Mekong Subregion Program Strategy 2030 Results Framework.*

Strategic Pillars and Programming Areas

Strategic Pillar 1: Regional Health Security

The vulnerability of the GMS to health security risks is widely acknowledged. The GMS is particularly vulnerable to infectious diseases due to its high biodiversity, frequent human to animal interactions, and rapid urbanization, which facilitate the spread of zoonoses and other pathogens. Additionally, cross-border trade, intensive livestock farming, weak health systems, and environmental degradation further contribute to the region's susceptibility to outbreaks and the rise of AMR; thus, it is critical for the GMS to align activities and technical areas that contribute to public health, preparedness, response, and resilience (footnote 4).

Programming Area 1.1: International Health Regulations Core Capacities

The International Health Regulations (2005) or IHR (2005) established the core capacity requirements of national health systems for preparing and responding to public health emergencies.[34] Supporting countries to implement and strengthen their health systems to manage outbreaks and prepare for a future pandemic is essential. The APHSAF builds on achievements, experiences, and lessons from almost 20 years of regional preparedness and response activities and provides a framework to support countries. The APHSAF considered ongoing global developments, including processes to amend IHR (2005), to develop and negotiate at the global level an international instrument for WHO on pandemic prevention, preparedness, and response (footnote 4). The APHSAF and IHR (2005) are key to the implementation of the HCS 2024–2030.

WHO set up an Intergovernmental Negotiating Body in December 2021 whose role was to draft what will become the new legally binding "pandemic instrument."[35] In May 2024, at the 77th World Health Assembly, all 194 WHO members approved a set of essential amendments to the IHR (2005) and pledged to finalize negotiations on a global pandemic agreement within a year. WHO states that these amendments will enhance global preparedness, surveillance, and response efforts for public health emergencies, including pandemics.[36]

Systematic tracking and analysis of environmental factors, such as monitoring air and water quality, changes in vector-borne diseases, and extreme weather events provide invaluable information for targeted interventions and building resilient health systems. Establishing a regional early warning and surveillance system for climate-related health risks and collaborating on air quality data to assess the impact of climate change would provide the GMS with an important evidence base for action.

By strengthening IHR core capacities, the region itself will be stronger, more robust, and better able to tackle future health security threats and provide an opportunity for the GMS countries to learn from each other through a series of regional exercises or drills and collaborative meetings on IHR. Existing

---

[34] The IHR (2005) is a legally binding agreement of 196 countries to build the capability to detect and report potential public health emergencies worldwide.

[35] WHO. 2022. Intergovernmental Negotiating Body.

[36] WHO. 2024. Seventy-Seventh World Health Assembly—Daily Update: 1 June 2024.

mechanisms and arrangements within the GMS will be leveraged, including through GMS-2030, to jointly build priority subregional capabilities (e.g., border control, field epidemiology, information technology and data). Assessing the financing gap needed to enhance IHR core capacities will be an important contribution of HCS 2024–2030. Showcasing the work of the WGHC through regional conferences, such as the annual Prince Mahidol Award Conference, will strengthen this collaboration.

Programming Area 1.2: Antimicrobial Resistance

Regional health security risks are compounded by increasing AMR, which poses a significant threat to health care as infections become more difficult to treat. In 2019, nearly 5 million deaths worldwide were linked to AMR, of these 1.27 million were directly attributable to antibiotic resistance, making AMR a primary cause of global mortality.[37] A 2010 study in Thailand found that more than 38,400 patients died with AMR hospital-acquired infections, and antimicrobial treatment for AMR infections in the same year cost $202 million, and $1.3 billion was the total cost associated with AMR-related morbidity and premature deaths.[38]

Controlling the emergence and spread of AMR pathogens is essential for effective disease treatment, reducing food safety and security risks, safeguarding the environment, and sustaining progress toward the SDGs (footnote 4). Tackling these challenges demands collaboration across animal, human, and environmental health sectors using One Health approaches. This includes surveillance and research, responsible antibiotic use for both human and animal health, and infection prevention and control measures.[39]

Essential for a successful response to AMR is to reinforce, strengthen, and utilize the existing AMR activities and regional networks, complementing the work being done by other partners, such as WHO. This will also provide an opportunity for the GMS countries to learn from each other and strengthen regional cooperation. For example, Thailand, a global leader in its One Health advancements, adopted and integrated a One Health approach for its National Strategic Plan on Antimicrobial Resistance.[40] Thailand hosts the regional base for the implementing agency of the Fleming Fund Regional Grants to address AMR. Cambodia has developed a comprehensive work plan for One Health, which aims to create an overarching One Health architecture focusing on three areas, including the reduction of AMR. Viet Nam's One Health Partnership Framework for Zoonoses, 2021–2025 includes initiatives on AMR.

---

[37] OECD and WHO. 2022. *Briefing Paper on Infection Prevention and Control: Addressing the Burden of Infections and Antimicrobial Resistance Associated with Health Care.*

[38] V. Thamlikitkul et al. 2015. Thailand Antimicrobial Resistance Containment and Prevention Program. *Journal of Global Antimicrobial Resistance.* 3. pp. 290–294.

[39] WHO defines One Health as an integrated, unifying approach that aims to sustainably balance and optimize the health of people, animals and ecosystems (source: WHO. One Health).

[40] G. Innes et al. 2022. *Enhancing Global Health Security in Thailand: Strengths and Challenges of Initiating a One Health Approach to Avian Influenza Surveillance. One Health.* 14. p. 100397.

Programming Area 1.3: Strengthen Communicable Disease Control Cross-Border Cooperation

Communicable disease control (CDC) systems are pivotal for safeguarding public health, encompassing a range of functions, including disease surveillance, early detection, investigation, response coordination, and public health education. International information-sharing and cooperation is done through the IHR (2005) and the national IHR focal points. Strengthening the mandate and capacities of CDC cross-border cooperation in line with the amended IHR (2005) is essential for improved health security. The WGHC will explore ways to strengthen information sharing on existing platforms, such as the Mekong Basin Disease Surveillance Foundation and ASEAN Emergency Operations Centre Network, to increase national and regional capabilities.

Enhancing cross-border CDC coordination and knowledge exchange through health emergency simulation exercises or drills, capacity building, mutual learning and strengthening regional digital platforms for sharing critical health information, early warnings, and surveillance data is key. The solutions for improved cross-border CDC coordination need to work at a national and subnational level; for example, during the pandemic, mutually accepted vaccine certificates were critical to facilitating cross-border travel and restarting tourism.

Strategic Pillar 2: Health System Strengthening Toward Universal Health Coverage

Strengthening the health system with an emphasis on equity and resilience is vital for achieving UHC and health security. This approach also supports broader socioeconomic advancement. According to UHC2030, it is the most effective and sustainable way to meet UHC and health security objectives.[41] GMS-2030 aims to accelerate the implementation of UHC, a critical regional public good, offering a chance for increased and more targeted investments in the core elements of health systems, particularly primary health care (PHC).

Service accessibility, availability, and individual acceptability play important roles in facilitating or hindering vulnerable populations, including older people's access to health care services.[42] Addressing these factors is crucial for achieving UHC, since it ensures everyone—regardless of their vulnerabilities—can receive the health services they need without facing financial hardship. By prioritizing the unique needs of these groups, health systems can reduce disparities, improve health outcomes, and promote equity, ultimately leading to a more inclusive and resilient health care system. For example, developing a regional telemedicine network could provide older people in remote areas with access to specialized care, demonstrating the importance of regional public goods in enhancing health care accessibility for vulnerable populations.

---

[41] UHC2030, formerly known as the International Health Partnership, is the global movement to build stronger health systems for UHC. The UHC2030 Secretariat is cohosted by WHO, the World Bank, and OECD, which support UHC2030's strategic vision and direction and promote collective action for universal health coverage. See UHC2030.org. *UHC 2030: Action on Health Systems, for Universal Health Coverage and Health Security*.

[42] M. Rosnu NS et al. 2022. Enablers and Barriers of Accessing Health Care Services Among Older Adults in South-East Asia: A Scoping Review. *Int J Environ Res Public Health*. 19 (12). p. 7351.

Programming Area 2.1: Access to Health Products

Access to high-quality health devices and products is essential for creating a foundation of consistency, quality, and responsiveness within health systems, including in primary health care. The GMS is heavily reliant on imports, and substantial investment in infrastructure and technological capabilities, including for local production, is necessary to enhance access to high-quality medical equipment and supplies. Established in 2014, the ASEAN Medical Device Committee was created to oversee the implementation of the ASEAN Medical Device Directive. This agreement aims to harmonize the regulatory framework for medical devices across the member states and was adopted to set technical standards, as well as to manage the registration and conformity of medical devices.[43] Developing and implementing these policies also promotes interoperability and improves the safety and efficacy of health care interventions.

The ASEAN has prioritized health care products, such as diagnostic tools, medicines, herbal remedies, and nutritional supplements, for the removal of technical trade barriers.[44] The HCS 2024–2030 will seek opportunities for public and private collaboration to increase availability and affordability of health products, including vaccines and pharmaceuticals.

Programming Area 2.2: Health Workforce and Infrastructure Development

Health security and health systems are mutually reinforcing, with strengthened functions in one leading to strengthened functions in the other (footnote 4). Equity is an important consideration in planning health services to ensure that all communities can access health care. Key to this is a health workforce—motivated, productive, and fit-for purpose and skilled—and appropriate health infrastructure. The HCS 2024–2030 will consider activities to strengthen the health workforce and explore opportunities to harness infrastructure advances and strengthen governance and regulatory infrastructure.

Aligning health workforce regulations across the GMS would allow for collaborative training programs and the mutual recognition of professional qualifications, enabling more seamless cross-border movement to address health care workforce shortages. Promoting standardized training and certification processes, developing processes for mutual recognition of qualifications and collaborative training programs, and seeking opportunities for cross country learning, e.g., through either regional centers of collaboration or through exchange, will further strengthen health systems and workforce development.

Programming Area 2.3: Service Delivery for All

As mentioned, achieving UHC requires addressing the health needs and equitable access to health care services for everyone, including migrants.[45] The challenges associated with the provision of migrant health are not new challenges for the GMS. There are a range of policies to protect the health of migrants, but migrant health is not just a matter of health—national security and economic concerns

---

43   ASEAN. *ASEAN Medical Device Directive*.
44   ASEAN. Standards and Conformance.
45   International Organization of Migration. 2019. *Information Sheet: Universal Health Coverage "Leave No Migrant Behind."*

are important factors influencing policies. There are some very pragmatic barriers; for example, linking individual identification of migrants to a provider for the whole year may be problematic when migrants change employers or move. The different needs of regular and irregular migrants should be considered, specifically with respect to health-seeking behaviors and barriers to service access.[46]

Regional UHC provides opportunities to advocate for migrant-inclusive health policies and explore ways to close the gap on insurance and the portability of insurance coverage. It could include activities to overcome some of the common barriers, such as duplication of health assessments and medical screening, facilitate continuity of care upon their arrival, and provide preventive and curative interventions (footnote 45). Implementation of the HCS 2024–2030 will look at ways to extend access to essential health services, policy coherence, and promoting financial risk protection for migrants.

Crosscutting Themes

The HCS 2024–2030 contains three crosscutting themes (gender, climate change, and digital health) that will be institutionalized across the strategic pillars.[47] The following discussion outlines the rationale for their selection and some of the programming opportunities that their inclusion might present.

Gender and Health

Gender equality is intrinsically linked to development, prosperity, and sustainability. Investing in the health and social workforce contributes to the achievement of UHC and health security, and, as revealed by the United Nations High-Level Commission on Health Employment and Economic Growth, these investments have a significant multiplier effect on economic growth and can contribute to maximizing women's economic empowerment and participation.[48]

Since 2000, GMS countries have progressed toward gender equality and all improved or maintained their Gender Inequality Index rankings in 2021. Despite progress, the region has not yet seen full and equal participation of women across social and economic spheres, nor have women benefited equally from the development initiatives to date. Many countries continue to grapple with high rates of adolescent pregnancy, high infant mortality rates, and maternal mortality rates; limited access to health care and reproductive services; and widespread gender-based violence. Women make up most of the health workers across the GMS and informal carers driven by entrenched gender norms.[49]

---

[46] Regular migration refers to the movement of persons within laws, regulations, or international agreements governing the entry into or exit from a state of origin, transit, or destination. Irregular migration refers to the movement of persons that takes place outside of regular migration channel (source: International Organization for Migration. 2019. International Migration Law No. 34—Glossary on Migration).

[47] The GMS-2030 proposed "innovative approaches" in six crosscutting areas and themes to guide the GMS Program, including (i) digital revolution, dialogue, knowledge sharing, and capacity building; (ii) private sector solutions; and (iii) GMS as an open platform, which are strong themes in the HCS 2024–2030.

[48] WHO. 2016, *Working for Health and Growth: Investing in the Health Workforce—Report of the High-Level Commission on Health Employment and Economic Growth.*

[49] ADB. 2022. *Greater Mekong Subregion Gender Strategy.*

The coronavirus disease 2019 pandemic exacerbated existing inequalities, especially gender disparities, and if these are not addressed, hard-fought gains for equality in the GMS will be lost (footnote 49). A 2022 study found that during the pandemic, intensified levels of preexisting widespread inequalities between women and men were seen. For example, women were more likely to report employment loss than men (26% vs. 20%) due to women working to care for others (ratio of women to men being 2:4). Women and girls were more likely than men and boys to drop out of school for reasons other than school closures. Women were more likely to report increased gender-based violence.[50]

While the health sectors in the GMS exhibit notable female participation, there remains a pressing need for gender-transformative policies to rectify disparities and dismantle obstacles hindering access to leadership positions. GMS-2030 has identified opportunities to advance gender equality in the GMS Program, and the GMS Gender Strategy, which was endorsed by the GMS countries in 2022, supports its implementation and complements the countries' efforts to enhance gender equality.[51]

Implementation of the HCS 2024–2030 will leverage those initiatives, and its activities will set specific targets to accelerate gender equality, including in health workforce development and leadership. It will support gender-responsive approaches to address gender issues and promote women's participation in the health sector.[52]

Climate Change and Health

Climate change is one of the seven long-term trends in GMS-2030. Its negative impact on health, and on the delivery of health care and quality health services, is well recognized. The Intergovernmental Panel on Climate Change states that climate change has already had diverse adverse impacts on human systems, including on water security and food production, health and well-being, and cities, settlements, and infrastructure.[53] WHO warns that climate change threatens the fundamental elements of good health—clean air, safe drinking water, a supply of nutritious food, and secure shelter. The impact has the potential to threaten decades of advancement.[54] During the 77th World Health Assembly, WHO members approved the first resolution on climate and health in 16 years.

In May 2024, a year after WHO's urgent call for global climate action to build resilient sustainable health systems,[55] its General Programme of Work 2025–2028 (GPW 14), which aims to address the growing health risks from climate change as one of its six strategic goals, was approved (footnote 28). Under the strategic objective of climate change and health, GPW 14 prioritizes two key areas: (i) strengthening climate-resilient health systems to protect people from the escalating health risks of

---

50 L. S. Flor et al. 2022. Quantifying the Effects of the COVID-19 Pandemic on Gender Equality on Health, Social, and Economic Indicators: A Comprehensive Review of Data from March 2020, to September, 2021. *The Lancet.* 399 (10344). pp. 2381–2397.

51 The Gender Strategy Implementation Plan 2030 will provide guidance on effective implementation of the GMS Gender Strategy, including areas of intersectionality, such as sexual orientation and gender identity.

52 A gender-responsive approach encompasses gender mainstreaming, informed by gender analysis, sex-disaggregated data, and consultation with women and vulnerable groups.

53 IPCC. 2022: *Summary for Policymakers. In: Climate Change 2022: Impacts, Adaptation and Vulnerability. Contribution of Working Group II to the Sixth Assessment Report of the Intergovernmental Panel on Climate Change.*

54 WHO. 2023. Climate Change and Health (accessed 16 October 2023).

55 WHO. 2023. WHO Issues Urgent Call for Global Climate Action to Create Resilient and Sustainable Health Systems (accessed 27 May 2024).

climate change; and (ii) advocating for and advancing lower-carbon health communities. According to WHO, these areas align with broader efforts to enhance primary health care, achieve UHC, and support climate resilience and mitigation initiatives.[56]

The One Health approach also offers a useful framework for addressing climate change and health, and the HCS 2024–2030 provides several avenues to support this area. These may include establishing a GMS climate change and health hub or network to cover a range of climate change-related areas. Such an initiative could focus on actions advancing implementation of national plans and ensuring that health is fully prioritized and integrated into national plans to fight climate change, provide technical support for policy reviews, and share good practices on climate change and health. For example, One Health could work to enhance information systems by integrating climate specific data; facilitating information sharing with a focus on developing skills in data analytics, modeling, and forecasting (e.g., floods and vector-borne diseases); considering how to improve or adapt health facilities impacted by climate change; recognizing or certifying "green facilities"; or collaborating on urban planning policies to develop cross-border healthy green cities.

Digital Health

The GMS countries have a common vision to integrate digital health information systems in all GMS health sectors and to optimize the use of digital technologies to strengthen the overall health system by 2030. Technological change and digitalization are also identified as one of the seven long-term, powerful local trends in GMS-2030 to encourage innovative strategies, harnessing the digital transformation to reshape economic sectors, such as health, for greater efficiency and inclusivity. In the GMS Digitalization Action Plan, health has been identified as a sector for priority collaboration.

The pandemic was a catalyst for the adoption of digital technologies in GMS countries. For example, in Cambodia, digital solutions, such as *KhmerVacc* (Cambodia's mobile app for vaccination registration) were deployed during the pandemic response. In Thailand, the Ministry of Public Health used *Mor Chana*, a mobile phone application, to support contact tracing efforts. In Viet Nam, a contact tracing application and a virtual health checkup platform called *Bluezone* were used. Under GMS-2030, collaborations with other sectors impacting health outcomes are being considered, including for digital health solutions and telemedicine to strengthen these information sharing platforms, thereby increasing national and regional capabilities, including for interoperability. HCS 2024–2030 will explore ways to expand GMS telemedicine services for treatment and to improve referral pathways.

---

56   WHO. 2024. WHO General Programme of Work 2025–2028 Prioritizes Climate Change and Health (accessed 26 June 2024).

Implementation Arrangements

During the consultation process for the first GMS Health Cooperation Strategy 2019–2023, the GMS countries had requested a comprehensive, coordinated, and proactive approach to address regional health issues (footnote 5), resulting in the establishment of the WGHC in 2019. The WGHC is a GMS governance platform that provides multilateral and bilateral coordination among the GMS countries. Before implementing the HCS 2024–2030, the terms of reference and composition of the WGHC and its Secretariat will be reviewed and adjusted. The WGHC will lead in the following for the HCS 2024–2030:

(i)   planning and delivery of health cooperation projects and activities;

(ii)   promoting knowledge sharing and information exchange on regional health issues through multiple channels;

(iii)   working with existing GMS networks and regional mechanisms;

(iv)   conducting coordination and consultation meetings; and

(v)   developing a regional health investment portfolio.

As the Secretariat of the GMS-2030, ADB will provide a grant for technical assistance (TA) to support the implementation of HCS 2024–2030 as it did in the first strategy. An output of the TA will be to support the operation and coordination of the WGHC and its Secretariat. This will include the establishment of a technical panel of experts with RCI experience, which the WGHC can agree to draw upon if technical feedback or advice is needed.

The GMS Program outlines a medium-term pipeline of priority projects across various sectors, including health, through its Regional Investment Framework (RIF), which is updated annually. In the GMS-2030, the RIF plays a pivotal role in identifying projects suitable for investment from public and private sources, with a strong focus on quality, sustainability, and promoting gender equality and social inclusion. The RIF pipeline is generated through WGHC inputs; broader conversations; and planning with GMS development partners, civil society organizations, and the private sector. Health cooperation projects stemming from the HCS 2024–2030 will continue to form an integral part of RIF. For a project to be included, projects must align with sector priorities and contribute to regional health cooperation outcomes by either (i) involving initiatives between two or more GMS countries or (ii) being a single-country initiative with clear benefits for other GMS countries.

Figure 2 presents a multilayered institutional framework of the GMS Program, which includes a Summit of Leaders every 3 years, ministerial conferences annually, and regular meetings of senior officials and sector working groups, including for health cooperation in the GMS countries (footnote 2).

Figure 2: Institutional Mechanism for Health Cooperation in the Greater Mekong Subregion

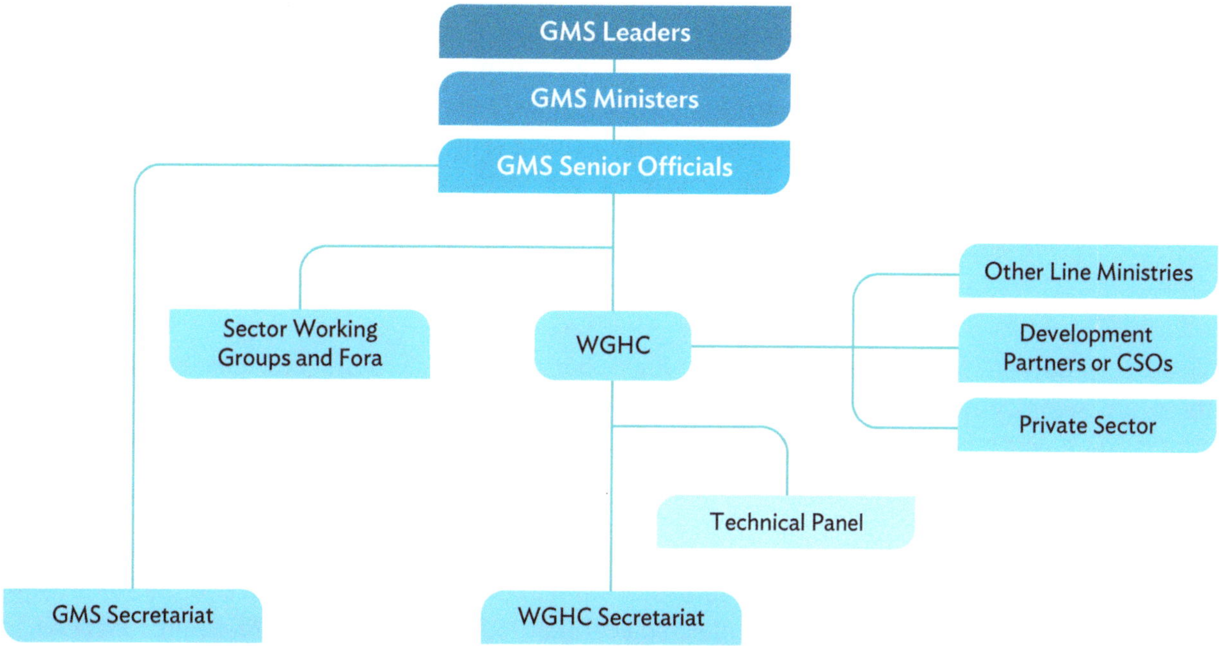

CSO = civil society organization, GMS = Greater Mekong Subregion, WGHC = Working Group on Health Cooperation.
Source: Asian Development Bank.

Monitoring Results

The proposed TA *Strengthening Regional Health Cooperation in the Greater Mekong Subregion (Phase 2)* will develop a design and monitoring framework of the HCS 2024–2030. In addition, a midterm review will be conducted in 2027 to identify where adjustments and adaptions are needed to ensure it meets its vision and objectives.

A wide range of stakeholders provided inputs to this strategy. This included the members of the GMS WGHC, stakeholders from the governments of GMS countries, development partners at both country and regional levels, United Nations agencies (e.g., WHO and International Organization for Migration), and civil society groups. Specific engagement with the private sector and local government authorities was sought to help broaden engagement.

Synergies with Other Sectors and Working Groups

The HCS 2024–2030 will continue to look for opportunities for cross-sector collaboration where there are significant common development benefits to health and another sector; for example, addressing environmental and climate change challenges by using green health infrastructure and technologies. It will also continue to explore opportunities for collaboration between the WGHC and ASEAN through the ASEAN Health Cluster Workplans and the Initiative for ASEAN Integration.

One Health is a good example of how intersector work in the GMS can be advanced. The approach, which considers human, animal, plant, and ecological health challenges, are all interconnected and has the potential to be transformational.[57] Addressing these challenges requires effective communication, cooperation, and joint efforts across various sectors, fields of expertise, and government levels. The One Health approach can provide multiple benefits. The approach is well understood by the countries of the GMS, which have been using it for several years. In May 2023, the GMS nations endorsed the ASEAN Leaders' Declaration on the One Health Initiative, committing to enhance and build multisector collaboration and coordination of One Health efforts among ASEAN member states. This includes creating connections with current or potential national mechanisms within these countries.[58]

---

[57] N. Habib et.al. Practical Actions to Operationalize the One Health Approach in the Asian Development Bank. *East Asia Working Paper Series.* No. 50. ADB.

[58] ASEAN. 2023. *ASEAN Leaders' Declaration on One Health Initiative.*

GMS-2030 intends to broaden the avenues for project investments and make it easier for the private sector and development partners to provide financing. The GMS Secretariat will promote combining policy reforms with private investments and public–private partnerships to unlock new funding sources, aiming to increase the positive effects of regional projects (footnote 2). The factors influencing health are wide-ranging, and many lie beyond the direct control of health-focused organizations. Public health policy is often determined by policies that guide actions beyond the health sector. Active cooperation and alignment with sectors beyond health care, such as environment, urban planning, tourism, and transportation is key for the effective implementation of the strategy. The GMS Program's sector working groups convene regionwide networks, which could be tapped to facilitate cross-sector collaboration and coordination. Various health impact assessment tools and methodologies have been developed in the past;[59] however, historically, the GMS Program has not seen many examples of joint projects that emphasize the synergies between health and the other sectors.

Role of the Private Sector and Development Partners

The health care needs of the GMS far outweigh what the public sector can provide. Despite the significant role the private sector plays in the economies of the GMS countries, the private sector's potential as a driver of inclusive economic growth remains largely unutilized, as noted in GMS-2030. Leveraging the knowledge and technical resources of the private sector, as well as its capital, is critical to achieving the ambitious health targets of the GMS countries. Primary health care is a driving force for advancing toward UHC. In 2019, modeling considered the level of additional investments needed to achieve a subset of PHC costs for each measure from the SGDs in 67 low- and middle-income countries, including the GMS. Between $200–$328 billion more is needed annually for PHC from 2020 to 2030.[60] Leveraging private sector capacity, investment, and innovation provides opportunities to address the issues of access, quality, and cost.

Development partners play a significant role in the health sectors of the GMS. They contribute to the region's efforts to improve health care access, quality, and outcomes, and addressing health disparities. In addition to ADB, partners include United Nations agencies (WHO, UNICEF, International Organization for Migration, and others); the Quadripartite (the Food and Agriculture Organization of the United Nations, United Nations Environment Programme, WHO, and World Organisation for Animal Health); as well as multilateral development banks (Asian Infrastructure Investment Bank, the World Bank, and Germany's KfW Development Bank). Bilateral development assistance from the governments of Australia, Japan, France, the PRC, the Republic of Korea, the United Kingdom, and the United States, as well as institutions in the European Union make a significant contribution.

Assistance is also provided through multilateral financing entities, such as the Global Fund to Fight AIDS, Tuberculosis and Malaria (the Global Fund) and Gavi, the vaccine alliance. The Global Fund's assistance is provided to each of the GMS countries, excluding the PRC, which had transitioned from Global Fund support in 2014. The assistance includes the Regional Artemisinin-Resistance Initiative

---

[59]   ADB. 2018. *Health Impact Assessment—A Good Practice Sourcebook*; WHO. 2018. Health in All Policies (accessed 26 October 2023).
[60]   K. Stenberg et al. 2019. Guide Posts for Investment in Primary Health Care and Projected Resource Needs in 67 Low-Income and Middle-Income Countries: A Modelling Study. *Lancet Glob Health*. 7 (11).

(RAI), which was established in 2013 to respond to malaria treatment resistance and eliminate *Plasmodium falciparum* malaria in the GMS. Between 2013 and 2023, the RAI has provided $585 million in grants, with its multisector Regional Steering Committee governing the grants.[61]

The Pandemic Fund created in September 2022 is the first multilateral financial mechanism aimed at providing multiyear grants to enhance pandemic preparedness in low- and middle-income nations.[62] This initiative is a partnership involving governments, the World Bank, WHO, United Nations bodies, multilateral development banks, global health organizations, philanthropies, and civil society groups. Its primary goal is to stimulate funding and foster coordination, with many projects focusing on regional cooperation and a One Health approach. In the GMS, Cambodia received a grant in the first round of the Pandemic Fund.

Role of Partnerships and Exchange

The HCS 2024–2030 will strengthen regional partnerships and exchange. It aligns with the action areas of the work plan for the Initiative for ASEAN Integration;[63] the technical networks mentioned earlier as well as the ASEAN University Network; Asia Partnership on Emerging Infection Diseases Research; Global Health Security Agenda; and One Health Universities Network. The WGHC platform serves to connect the efforts of these networks with the Regional Investment Framework and potential sources of funding from development partners. The strategy will explore other opportunities for the GMS countries to learn from each other and establish centers of excellence or collaboration. For example, the PRC has proposed the establishment of an "ASEAN Plus China" Women and Children's Health Cooperation Center, and Thailand has proposed field epidemiology training to support improved surveillance and outbreak response in the GMS.

Risk Management

The HCS 2024–2030 may face various risks and challenges during its implementation. These risks could include health-related threats (i.e., another pandemic), political and economic challenges, and operational difficulties. Specific risks might include the following:

(i)   **Climate change and environmental risks.** Climate change-related events, such as floods and changing disease vectors, could exacerbate health risks and strain health care systems.

(ii) **Emerging health threats.** New and unexpected health threats, such as novel pathogens or drug-resistant infections, may require rapid response and adaptation of the strategy.

61   The Global Fund. 2023. RAI Regional Steering Committee (accessed 10 January 2024).
62   World Bank. 2023. The Pandemic Fund.
63   ASEAN Secretariat. 2020. *Initiative for ASEAN Integration (IAI) Work Plan IV (2021–2025)*.

(iii) **Competition for resources.** The allocation of resources including for health care personnel may compete with health priorities.

(iv) **Economic shocks.** Economic downturns or financial crises could impact government budgets and the availability of funds for health programs.

(v) **Global health governance.** Changes in global health governance and international funding priorities may influence the level of support and coordination for regional health cooperation initiatives.

The Secretariat of the WGHC will lead the ongoing risk assessments and develop risk mitigation plans to maintain flexibility to adapt to changing circumstances. By proactively addressing these risks, the strategy can become more resilient and better equipped to achieve its vision and objectives.